Shape Your Style

Guide to Confidently Dress

Any Body Shape

To my mom Deena and dad Timothy,

Thank you for giving me life, encouraging me to follow my dreams, and allowing me the space to grow and be creative. I hope you are proud of the woman I am becoming each day as this is only the beginning.

-Love your babygirl,

Aaliyah

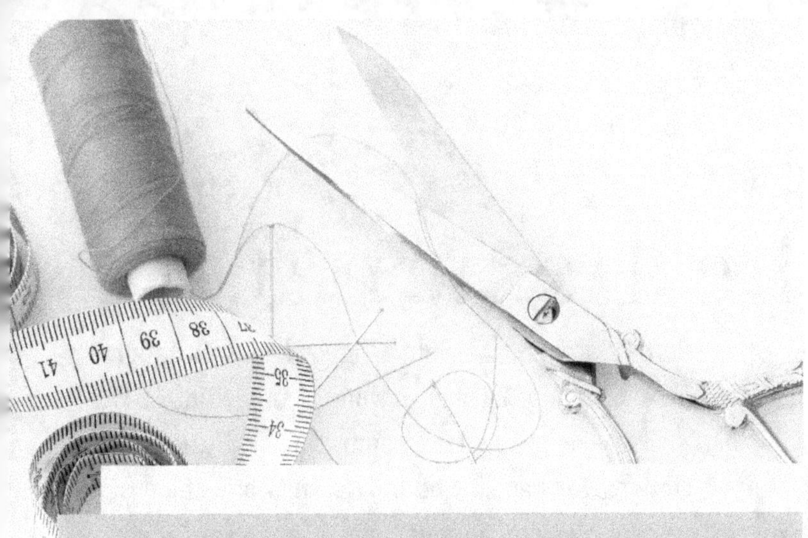

TABLE OF
CONTENTS

the Designer

Residing in North Carolina, Aaliyah Wright is a self taught fashion designer who started her sewing journey in 2017. Evolving her skills as a seamstress completing alterations on store bought clothing for herself and others, then branching off to begin experimenting with various fabrics and creating her own pattern pieces from scratch. Today, Aaliyah has been repeatedly invited to be featured in numerous fashions shows all over the Carolinas, she has multiple viral videos on social media of sewing tutorials and fashion tips, all while creating custom formal gowns for special occasions including proms, galas, birthdays and even weddings!

CONTACT ME

Email :
aalichaw@gmail.com

Website :
www.aalichaw.com

Social Handle:
@aalichaw

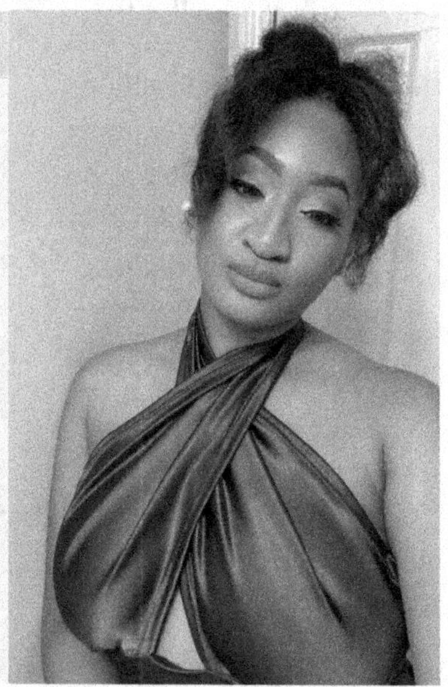

Intro: My Intention

"I could never wear that… " is probably the most common statement I hear from people. Especially when they see someone else's outfit, or when they themselves are encouraged to try something new to wear.

As a seamstress and fashion designer, I can't help but cringe every time I hear this. I know that more often than not, this couldn't be further from the truth. Fashion is all about expression. It is an art form that is certain to look different for everyone. To say that you could never wear something, is to say that you can never express yourself freely. I don't know about you, but to me that sounds like such a painful and unfulfilling life to live.

Before we get into styles and bomb outfits, I have to make something very clear. There is one thing so crucial that everyone needs to have first. It's something that can't be bought in stores, and it can't fully be taught either. If you lose it, the results are detrimental to you and your overall success in life. In my years of experience, I can honestly say that the key to executing any flawless look or opportunity comes down to just one simple thing. C O N F I D E N C E ! Now I know what you're thinking. "That is so cliché… I did NOT come here for lesson in confidence. I came here for the fits!" Trust me, I get it! And I'll get to that part, I promise. But I would be remiss not to include confidence in this book. I built my entire company based off of this sole concept. First, in order to empower myself as a young black woman, then to empower the other beautiful women around me. Although I do have tips for the fellas, women get a front seat at this table.

Shockingly, research shows that over 70% of women struggle with confidence, body image, and self worth. Specifically, women of color in America struggle even more so. A study done by *Dove* in 2017 surveyed over 10,000 women across the globe. The survey reported that only 4 percent of women worldwide considered themselves beautiful. Part of this may be due to the previous beauty standards celebrated in high places like Hollywood. These standards were being based solely from the looks of European women beginning back in the 17th century. To put this into perspective, this was over 400 years ago. Today what is still celebrated the most is pale skin, pencil thin, and long straight hair blowing in the wind. Although beautiful, it's not very inclusive.

Iconic fashion shows like New York Fashion Week didn't have a plus size label walk the runway until 2013. Fenty Beauty made history in the makeup industry just in 2017, launching with a broader range of shades to include darker skin tones. Laws like the CROWN Act protecting natural hair from discrimination weren't even established until 2019. It is even rare to see any aged women portrayed as beautiful in anything other than commercials for a new medication. Crazy, right? And we haven't even touched on the issues women face at the workplace or in relationships. Although we have come a long way in changing the beauty standards, we still have a long way to go while women continue to pick up the pieces of their shattered self esteem.

     While well-put together outfits may not directly solve these or the many other issues women face, this book is my attempt to give women a starting place. A safe place to begin gaining your power back. As we all know, when you look good, you feel good. Whether male or female, my goal is to guide you to feel good from the inside out. Maybe this is the start of a new you. Maybe the outfit you wear is the only thing you feel you have control over right now in your life. Maybe you are still getting used to the body that you have today versus the one you had years ago. Either way, you are welcome here. You are safe here. I invite you to feel free and get comfortable while you enter into this space where I share some of my own vulnerable moments. I'll touch on some of the many times that I myself have struggled with confidence, self worth and my fashion sense. Then, I'll go over exactly what I did to slowly but surely grow into my own level of success in these same areas. Walk with me through this journey of how I built confidence starting from the inside out, then one outfit at a time. And how regardless how your life may look or feel right now, you can do the same!

Fashion in Practice

How you carry yourself in an outfit can really make or break a look. When you feel secure about who you are, you're more likely to show your personality through your style no matter where you go. Also, when you feel good about your appearance, you will probably dress in ways that enhances your favorite features of yourself. This in turn makes you feel the most comfortable and confident. The opposite is also true. When you don't feel secure or positive about yourself, you're likely to shrink yourself in rooms or hide your full self behind your clothes. You may even neglect certain self care practices such as routine grooming, scheduled down time for yourself, and connecting with those around you.

Even the best outfits can be ruined if you slouch with your arms folded when you walk, or have to constantly keep tugging at a piece of clothing you are wearing, or if you feel so awkward that you just end up throwing on an ill-fitting sweater or jacket to cover it all up. These are all examples of negative body language. What you are subconsciously telling others around you is "I'm uncomfortable." "I'm unsure of myself." "I don't feel worthy." And If you're not careful, you will actually start to be treated this way by those around you in response. Even though it may not be something you or those around you consciously do on purpose, energy responds to energy. The type of energy you put out about yourself is the same energy you will attract back to you. This is why confidence is key!

The textbook definition of confidence is the firm trust or belief that you can rely on someone or something. In this instance, we use it to have a firm belief and trust in yourself when it comes to your fashion choices. It can even be the assurance you have in your own capabilities to get things done in a way you desire. But how exactly do you get confident? If you are anything like me, I have always wondered how confident people got that way. Where they born with it? Is it a muscle that can be trained to grow over time? Admittedly, I've struggled with confidence from elementary school all the way up until after graduating college. That's right. Even as a full-grown adult paying my own bills, I still struggled.

I was a shy kid. Never said too much, if I ever said anything at all when going into a new environment. My mom would lecture me saying "How can you be shy? You are a child of the most high God!" I remember thinking to myself after her long sermons, "But what does that even mean? And how does that cure shyness?" We didn't have much money and because my mom lived majority of my childhood stressed trying to make ends meet, things like retail therapy, vacations, or going out to eat seemed like a far off luxury. My clothes were often hand me downs given to us from church or if we were lucky, new and gifted to us by my cool aunts. Sometimes they were worn by my mom first, then my older sister, then me. The times we had a car were sporadic, so walking and catching the bus became the norm. Almost every year or so, we would bounce around from apartment to apartment or lived with a different family member because we couldn't afford rent.

Every now and then, I even remember mom would order a couple of cheeseburgers from the fast food dollar menu and cut them in half. This was to make it stretch between me and my siblings. She rarely saved anything for herself to eat.

As a result, I always felt out of place and unworthy. I started to visibly see the differences between me and other girls around my age at the time. I would go to school and see them having the nicer clothes with the aroma of fancy smelling lotions or perfumes filling the air as they walked by. All while talking about how their family tried a new restaurant last night or where they went for their family vacation or making plans with their friends on what time they would meet at the mall or movie theater later that day. Then when school was out, they would simply walk out to the parking lot where their parents pulled up in a shiny car and drove off. I on the other hand, would then adjust my backpack straps to prepare for my 20 to 30 minute walk home, depending on how heavy my book bag was that day.

Now the walking wasn't too bad. I liked the time to myself, although the winters in Ohio can be brutal. And my clearly out of style and second hand clothes did in fact keep me covered and from getting sick. Maybe it was my immaturity or lack of knowledge at the time, but I just couldn't figure out how being a "child of God" was supposed to make me stand up tall and justify me not being able to have what the other girls had. I had begun the habit of comparing myself to others and would feel instantly ashamed and embarrassed at the drastic differences I would find. Looking back, I can now see that a lot of the resilience I have today stems from my mother's strength during these times where we didn't have much.

But because I started comparing myself to the other girls,

my confidence plummeted.

Regardless of my mother's best efforts to convince

me, none of the talks seemed to work. This continued for

years. Eventually, I took matters into my own hands and

began my journey of learning what self confidence meant

and looked like to ME. Over time I learned many practices

to boost my self esteem but back then, my first order of

business was to start with my second hand clothes. Before

I learned how to sew, I would twist and tie clothes in

different ways so that it looked what I felt was completely

different from when my big sister or mom wore it. The fact

that I created a new look from an old one and could wear it

proudly at school definitely gave me a new perspective on

fashion. Little did I know, this would be the genesis of my company AALICHAW Designs years later.

I was introduced to sewing in middle school. The class was called Home Economics and the assignment for that week was to hand sew a pillow. I should have known then that I was interested in sewing, because of course my pillow was the talk of the class! While everyone else's pillow was the traditional two large squares sewn together on all 4 sides, mine was far more elaborate. I cut out each letter of my name in various colors of pink fabric and hand stitched them on my front square. Then for the back square, I cut out diagonal pieces of those same pink fabrics and organized them from light to dark, for an ombré effect. After sewing each stripe together in order, I then trimmed the edges to make a perfect square. Then finally, I sewed those two squares together.

Unfortunately by the end of the next week, I didn't think too deeply about sewing anymore. I knew that when I left school at the end of the day, sewing wasn't going to bring food in the house, pay the bills or relieve the stress my mom experienced daily. It wasn't a priority. I viewed it as just part of the assignment and was only trying to get a good grade. That's it. However, this was the catalyst for me to get comfortable with sewing and this confidence with a needle came in handy for my future fashion projects.

It wasn't until later in my adult life that my creativity fully sparked again. By this time, I was living with my big sister Morgan while in college and working at the hospital where we lived. Life was in full effect and I now had a deeper understanding of how easy it is to get sucked into the stressful cycle I watched my mom endure. Caught in the loop of working only to pay bills. I had just gotten home from work exhausted from the day and just wanting to wind down. As I kicked off my shoes and threw my purse down on the couch, I grabbed the TV remote and turned it on to a random channel. I hoped to tune out the noise in my head with the noise from the TV. I plopped myself down on the couch, closed my eyes, and took a deep breath. When I open my eyes, I noticed the channel I had randomly selected, was showing the hit series *Project Runway*. Fixated on the screen, all I could think to myself was "I could do that… I CAN do that." By the time my imagination landed back on earth, it was already dark. I had been watching *Project Runway* for four hours straight.

The very next day I went to the nearest Walmart to buy the nicest looking machine I could afford. Funny enough, the one I liked had a label on the box that read,

Project Runway Limited Edition. "Okay God. I hear you." I

thought to myself, then brought it home. I rummaged

through my closet for clothes that I knew didn't fit quite like

how I wanted them to and started tinkering. Next thing you

know, I'm buying fabric by the yard at my local craft store

and started tinkering with that too. The projects that went

well, I took pictures of and posted them on my social

media. At the time, I wasn't really expecting much

interaction from these posts. I was just happy that I could

create something with my own hands. From there, word

spread quickly that I could sew. Just from those few posts,

people started asking if could I make alterations on their

clothes too.

I hesitated at first, because I didn't feel completely ready to be at the mercy of someone else's opinion of my work. This was still a new hobby for me and I hadn't quite gotten the hang of it yet. Because I had been asked so many times by different people, and with the encouragement from Morgan, eventually I caved. Slowly I'd grown a small number of repeated clients including Morgan. Soon after, I took the leap and quit my job after graduating college and pursued my sewing business full-time. Completing successful alterations on other peoples clothing gave me the sense of accomplishment that I had back when I made my first pillow. I came to the conclusion that I could make the same, if not more, income that I had working at the hospital if I poured my full self into this new found passion.

After a few months of doing this and driving Uber between projects, Morgan came home from work one day and said that she found out there was a local seamstress in town. The seamstress had been overwhelmed with work and was desperately looking for help. Morgan suggested that I to go to the seamstress shop to see if they would be willing to take me in. I liked the idea and knew that it would be beneficial for me to see someone successfully doing what I wanted to do but on a larger scale. So I made my way to the seamstress shop, introduced myself to the owner, and explained how I am new at sewing and interested in fashion. With excitement, the owner said she'd be happy to have me. She hired me on the spot, but noted that she wouldn't be sure if she could pay me right away. I was only learning through trial and error on my own and knew that the knowledge I would be receiving from being there would pay me soon enough, so I agreed to

start the unpaid internship for the experience.

After I joined the shop, it felt like things were falling

into place one by one. I told my small number of clients

that I worked at an official shop now so they could come

see me there anytime they had something for me to work

on. At this point because I had beaten her to the shop

every morning, the owner gave me my very own key to

open the store myself. Soon, the work that piled up was

quickly finished and rotated back out to the clients. She

taught me many alteration techniques and always

reviewed my work to make sure it was a clean finish. I was

learning so much about the business side of sewing from

inside a real life store front. Plus, since the workload had

now been lifted, we had time to tinker around with different

scrap fabrics and clothing designs for fun. This was a

crucial time for me because it was then that the owner

observed my work and noted, "I think formal gowns are

your thing!" I had found my niche.

I even got to make outfits for the owner herself

which she wore with the biggest smile to a couple of her

business events. With me as her plus one to a few of the

local Chamber of Commerce business meetings, she

would introduce me to the other business owners boasting

"This is my lovely assistant!" and "I brought my protégé

with me!" We brainstormed on T-shirt ideas to sell as

merchandise in the shop lobby to generate passive income

and started posting more on the owners social media page

to promote the store. The shop was doing so well that the

owner was even able to rent out the neighboring office

space to expand our working area. The owner was also

able to get involved with the local high schools so that

students interested in fashion could get school credit for internship by coming to the shop a couple days out of the week. I also got the opportunity to step into a managerial role for the first time and oversee a few of the students projects. By now, the owner was able to pay me a little here and there for my work along with treating me to lunch everyday. In order to get a consistent paycheck each week, the owner then partnered with the local employment center to start getting me paid for being there. Now I started to get paid well and regularly for doing work that I love! It felt surreal. Most people would tell you that it's just a pipe dream to get paid doing what you love and everyone hates their job because that's just how life goes. Here I was, proving that myth totally wrong.

About six months in being an intern, things started to change. There was a period of time where the owner had to be out for a couple of weeks, so she trusted me to

open the shop in her place. Because I had already been

doing this unofficially, I felt sure I could handle it. She

assured me that I would still have help as she would send

one of her family members, whom I had now started to

become close with, to check in on me during store

hours. Although they weren't exactly well versed with a

sewing machine, I did enjoy the company.

The first week of the owners absence went well. I

had been doing my work as usual and being sure not to

take on any projects I felt uncomfortable with. I feared that

I may mess up a garment and give the owner's shop a bad

reputation. My comfort zone at the time was tailoring pants

and skirts. I mastered shortening pants and skirts that

were too long and occasionally taking them in at the waist

or leg if they were too wide. Anything besides that, I would let the customer know when the owner would be returning

and that she would handle that garment herself as soon as

she could. Their response was always something along the

lines of "Thats fine! It's no rush at all. Thanks!" But by the

second week of opening the shop by myself, there was a

shift. When one of the owner's family members came in,

they started to ask strange questions.

"Is everything alright at home?" "You know if you

need any help here you can call one of us right?", one of

the family members would ask. A day or so would go by

and the same questions were asked again, but by a

different family member. "What is going on?", I thought to

myself. Had I been doing a bad job? Did somebody

complain about me? I hadn't heard anything. I know I

made sure to avoid any projects I didn't feel 100%

comfortable working on. Only tailoring pants and skirts. No wedding gowns, no prom gowns, no men's suit jackets. So why were they asking me these questions? I figured I was just being paranoid and that the owner and her family was only making sure I felt comfortable. However, when I went to collect my weekly check from the local employment center, my suspicions grew.

My career coach sat me down before handing me my check for the week saying she wanted to talk for a minute. "The owner just left here awhile ago. She spoke with me saying that she was concerned about you," my career coach began. "Concerned?" I said confused both at the surprise visit from the owner, and why she shared these supposed concerns with my career coach and not me directly. "I haven't heard anything.. I did think it was strange that her family members kept asking me if I felt okay or if I needed help." My career coach then started to lay out a number of complaints that the owner shared with her about me, just moments before I walked in. Apparently, the owner felt that I had poor customer service and said my work wasn't any good, among other complaints.

This took me by surprise because I genuinely thought I was doing well. I knew I was a beginner with a lot to learn, but I also knew I brought value to her store. Look at how much we accomplished so far. I was working so hard and hadn't heard any of these complaints from her before now. I had been there for months. On top of the fact that I hadn't heard any of these complaints from any customers or the family members the entire time I was handling the shop by myself. Anytime someone came to pick up their garments, I would show them the work that I did, they paid with a smile and instructed me to say hello

to the owner when she returned. That was it.

"So she hasn't said anything to you?" My career

coach asked. "No.." I replied, now kind of hurt to learn that

there had been private conversations about me when I

wasn't around. First between the shop owner and her

family members, and now with my career coach. I was the

only one out of the loop. I also started to worry that this

would affect my pay from the employment center. I had

quit my job for this after all. Had I made a bad decision in

quitting my job for a fantasy? My anxiety went through the

roof.

After assigning me a number of customer service

and business ethics courses online, my career coach

advised that all three of us should have a group meeting so

that everyone would be on the same page. This meeting wasn't for another week or so and I was still expected to open up the shop. I started to feel more and more uneasy about working there. Shortly after that, the shop owner returned to the store and continued business as usual. Except now it felt as if there was this invisible wall between us. She still never brought up the complaints that she discussed previously with my career coach, so I didn't bring them up either. Surely it was just a misunderstanding.

Days later, one of the repeat customers I had before I started at the shop called my cell phone. I'd done work for him a few times previously on my own but after learning I was at the shop, he came to drop off more work for me there. "I felt that you should know because I thought it was strange. I came to pick up the work you did for me and that woman started talking about you and your work. I looked at your work myself and I didn't see a problem. I don't think she knew I was one of your regulars before coming here," he said.

It hurt. I looked up to the shop owner. She taught me so much. I thought I was doing well, but according to her rumors, clearly I wasn't. And now I knew for sure that intentional secret conversations are still being had about me and I can't even defend myself. I didn't know what to do. I still liked doing the work, but felt like maybe all this was just a pipe dream after all. I continued my work as usual, and said nothing. The little girl from middle school who felt unworthy and out of place had returned. Along with being timid, she hated confrontation. All I felt I could do was count down the days until it was time for the group meeting with hopes that all three of us would surely come to a better understanding.

A couple days before our meeting, the owner was checking behind my work, as she would usually do. However on this particular day, she finally said what I think she had been wanting to say for a while. "I appreciate you being here and helping out, but your work SUCKS.. " she blurted out. My heart shattered. I'm not sure what she said after that because the only thing that kept ringing in my head was "your work sucks….Your work SUCKS…. YOUR WORK SUCKS…." I remained silent, still working at my desk until closing time. My dream work environment had now turned in to what felt like a prison with the owner's harsh words being the ball and chain strapped to my ankles preventing me to move. After finally closing the shop that day, I drove home, curled up in my bed and cried.

The next day I called out. This was the first time I hadn't shown up at the store since I'd started. Instead, I went to see my career coach at the employment center to explain what happened the day before. "We don't have to waste any time with the group meeting because I'm not going back there. I'm quitting" I said. "Well, the intern program we have you on is for 12 weeks total and you only have two weeks left. You'd be giving up free money..." My career coach said, noticing I wasn't moved by her words. "Tell you what, let's have the meeting first and then see how you feel afterwards, Okay?" Reluctantly, I agreed, but my mind was already made up. I was ready to quit sewing and never look at another sewing machine again. After all, this wasn't just some stranger on the street commenting on my work. This was my teacher. The person who called out my niche before I even could see it myself. She knew what I was capable of so her words must have been true, right? If so, I felt there was no need for me to continue in this field.

Finally the day came for the long awaited three-way meeting, but I didn't say a word. My career coach did majority of the talking expressing the concerns that she had heard from the both of us individually. She then asked if she left anything out or if we wanted to add to what she shared. The owner took this opportunity to apologize for her "choice of words", but the apology didn't stop the haunting moment from continuing to ring in my head. I thought about how relieved she was when I introduced myself to her the first day I walked in. I thought about the day she gave me my own store key. I thought about how fast the work she was so overwhelmed with was cleared out with my help. I thought about the business meetings she brought me to. The outfits I'd made for her. The t-shirt

ideas I came up with. The office expansion. The marketing

I had done. The additional clients I brought to the store.

The months I worked for free before the internship started.

I wondered just how much income I must have helped her

bring into the shop all for it to be summed up with those

three piercing words. Noticing I had been silent the entire

time, my career coach asked did I have anything I wanted

to share or add. I responded with a quiet but sure "No."

They decided I should stay the last two weeks of the intern

program I was on, but after that I knew I was done. I didn't

hear about any complaints after that.

After the program ended, I returned my shop key

and went to collect my last check from the employment

center. I briefly started thinking about getting another 9 to

5 job and go back to driving Uber in the meantime. My

career coach told me to let her know if I wanted her to look up any other businesses they were partnered with, but because I was so broken up inside, I thanked her and declined. I just wanted to be left alone for awhile in fear that my next boss may break my spirit even further with more harsh words. I was also prepared to sell my sewing machine. Right when I decided on giving up sewing completely, I got a message from my Facebook page. "Hello, Aaliyah! My name is Sheila and I have been following you for some time online. Your work is amazing! I was wondering if you would be interested in being a part of my fashion show in Charlotte, NC. If so, give me a call and we can work out the details!" They say when one door closes, another one opens. You see how God works?

If that wasn't enough to begin mending my self-esteem, the shop owner later reached back out to me. She said work had piled up again due to prom season and she was wondering if I would be available to help her. She even noted that she'd be able to pay me herself this time. Respectfully, I declined and said I was overwhelmed myself with a fashion show I was preparing for. If I'm being completely honest, it felt so good to let her know that I had moved on without her. This turned out to be the very first fashion show I've ever done, and built the confidence that I have to take on the many shows I've done thus far. As time went by, I was able to see past my hurt feelings from being at the shop. Today, the shop owner and I are still in contact and even support each other's work regularly.

I share these stories not to shame or embarrass anyone, but to use my own experiences as an example. These were all significant moments in my life that shaped who I've become today along with my fashion sense. The experiences compounded with each other and broadened my overall outlook on life and business. Both the good and the not so good. One of my good mentors Tiffany Aliche once said "nothing you experience is wasted."

Self-esteem, fashion, and life are all a journey. The three intersect in such meaningful ways that shape our sense of self, how we interact with others, and the life stories we create for ourselves. You change and grow. It's in our nature. Being able to use our past experiences as fuel and a measuring point for the future is probably one of our greatest superpowers as humans. It also takes continuous work. You constantly reshape and mold yourself. After these and future events, my confidence was still shaky, but improving. There were many highs and many lows. Throughout these life fluctuations, even my closet reflected the inconsistencies of how I felt along the way.

After I left the shop and experienced my very first fashion show, I wasn't exactly sure of what to do next or who I was as an individual. Although I knew I wanted to be have a successful fashion brand someday, I didn't know where to start, what styles my brand would represent, or who my target audience would be. There was no business plan, no LLC, not to mention I still had issues finding my own style within my closet. During this time, I was still in the beginning stages of becoming a young adult.

Back when we first moved from Ohio to North Carolina, I was a freshman in high school. I spend three years in Charlotte making friends, learning the new city and began building my resources that I knew I would need by graduation. My teachers, counselors, and friends at school played the largest part in this. I stayed in the top 10% of students when it came to academics, signed up for driver's education, applied for local scholarships and grants while visiting colleges in the area, and I was well known and high ranked in JROTC for all three years. That meant if I chose to go into the service after graduation, I would start off with a higher-ranking than those who weren't in JROTC in high school.

However, towards the end of my junior year in high school, my mom decided that it was a good idea for us to move again. Still in North Carolina, but in a city about an hour away. This meant I would be starting at a new school again, but this time during my senior year of high school. The most important and meaningful year for a teenager. I was livid. All my plans, my friends, my resources were about to be blown away. Everything that I worked to build up was based on me living in Charlotte. A relocation meant that I no longer qualified for those scholarships for college, drivers ed, or the JROTC promotion that required 4 consecutive years. I had to start over all the work I did within those three years in the new location, but with only one year to work with AND as the new girl in a small city. And that's only if the same resources were available where we were moving to. It was then that I started to slip into depression.

Fast forward and somehow, I managed to graduate high school in the new city, then community college, and worked that 9 to 5 job at the hospital before I started working at the shop. But now, I felt lost. None of those things seemed fill the void within me. None of that taught me who I was or how the world actually works. Plus, I had just experienced my first gut punch of what entrepreneurship can feel like from the internship. There were still pieces within me that missed my friends and I ruminated about what my life would have looked like had we never moved away from Charlotte. I even began to feel distant from my family back in Ohio. Birthdays, graduations, and holidays passed and my cousins who I felt so close to when we were kids, were now full adults like me and some even were parents now.

I also didn't feel like I had any real guidance. My dad lived hundreds of miles further south in an entirely different state ever since I was young so I always felt he was out of reach. And by this time, my mom decided to move again hundreds of miles north about a year or two after my high school graduation. It was a lot going on at once. It felt strange. Here I was clearly over the drinking age and still didn't have a clue about life or myself. On top of the fact that I just came out of a romantic relationship. I share all this to put into perspective the combination experiences that influenced my confidence to mirror a warped and withered version of myself. I remember talking to Morgan and expressing that I felt I was in a "quarter-life crisis." This was the very first time I had the chance to just look around and observe my life and others without my parents, a job, school or any other possible filter.

As a result, I felt that I didn't really know much, have much, or do much of anything meaningful. I felt alien on the very earth I was born on. This feeling of being mismatched in life bled out into my closet and clothing

choices. I didn't really know what I liked or exactly what

look I was going for. I already wasn't comfortable shopping

because it was a rare occasion growing up. I would either

avoid shopping all together or find myself ordering bulks of

clothes online, but only wearing two or three of those

things. And even those still didn't fit quite right. After I

spent majority of the time feeling unhappy with my life and

uncomfortable in my clothes, I decided it was time to

reshape my closet and my lifestyle.

It was when my sister and I both hit rock bottom

and struggled to make ends meet that I started to make a

change. We ended up having to move again and again. My

childhood seemed to be repeating itself in my adulthood

and that scared me. This was the turning point for me

where I started to look for answers. It was here that I

formed what I call my mental fitting room. You know how when you go shopping and you want to try on what you picked out to see if it works for you? I did the same thing but for my mind. I got sick and tired of being sick and tired so I needed to try out some new ways of thinking and living to see what works for me.

When I looked around seeking advice, that's when I started to realize many people struggled with confidence and living a live that was meaningful to them, too. Although I did feel less alone hearing the life stories of others, I also felt it just didn't make sense how so many people around me struggled to find solutions to the same problems. It was the blind leading the blind. I decided it was time to take a deep dive to understand my internal struggles and how to overcome them. My lifestyle and fashion sense was at stake.

The Fitting Room

In school, my favorite subject was science. I loved to figure out how and why things worked the way that they do. This situation was of no exception. At first, I started googling random but related topics about building self esteem, lifestyle, beauty, and fashion. As I spiraled down many rabbit holes all at once, I quickly realized it was difficult to organize and connect all the pieces of the information I was learning. Where should I start? What could I work on right now? What was the most important? Then I came across a psychology chart titled "Maslow's

Hierarchy of Needs." This chart's most popular illustration was in the shape of a pyramid. It listed what Abraham Maslow, an American psychologist from Brooklyn, New York in the mid 1900s, discovered what the needs of humans are in order to have an overall sense of well-being. Stay with me, because this all comes full circle when it relates to fashion. We are working from the inside out, remember?

As I reviewed this pyramid of needs from the bottom up, it was clear that a lot of what the illustration showed that humans needed in order to have a good sense of well being, I didn't have as an adult. These needs also weren't consistently maintained in my childhood either. I now identified where the gaps were in my life and could name the exact areas I needed to improve. Confronting these areas in turn would stimulate lasting confidence within myself, then be reflected back out through my fashion sense. Although the different stages of the pyramid are related and can be addressed simultaneously, for me I took it one level at a time. As I began to accomplish one level, my confidence grew which fueled my motivation to confront the next level head on.

The first level, at the very bottom of the pyramid, Maslow listed that this is the foundation of what all humans need in order to physically survive. These are the basics of what keeps us from going extinct as a species. This portion of the pyramid is called the Physiological Needs. This includes air, water, food, sleep, your reproductive system, shelter and yes even clothing. At this stage, the clothing isn't concerned with fashion just yet, but it is required in order to regulate your body temperature from the outside elements. I like to call this stage Survival Mode, because without these basic needs being met, it is difficult to care about much else. Therefore, your self-esteem, confidence, creativity, and even empathy for others may seem to be mentally turned off in this stage. It my sound silly or obvious that these needs are to be met first, but you'd be surprised how a lack in any one of these areas can have life long effects on a person's confidence if not addressed.

For example, because keeping food in the house was such a sacrifice for us growing up, it became a habit to completely clean my plate when it was time to eat. If we wasted anything, we'd get in big trouble for it. I also only learned to shop for and cook foods that were cheap and/ or able to stretch for days at a time. I also got used to ill-fitting clothes. Even though I didn't particularly like the clothes mom got us, I knew it was all we had. I just had to wait until I grew out of the too big clothes, then I could get

something else. And as far as shelter, moving from place to

place every year or so almost trained me to master

detachment. Because I knew I most likely wasn't going to

stay in one place for long, I made little to no effort to

connect with people around me. I would disassociate

myself from others and became timid when approached.

Each and every one of these traits carried into my

adulthood. When I started noticing that other people

behaved differently than I did when it came to these areas,

I was often amazed. I liked the sense of freedom I saw

people operating in and wanted to feel that for myself too.

So now that I knew what my weak areas were in this first

level of the pyramid, I tacked them first. Shelter, food and

clothing. It helped that I was living with my big sister and

we split the bills between us. This took care of most areas

in this first stage in the pyramid. My sister and I bought
each other food often and even went out to dinner each
week or so. This broke the feeling of lack that we had
growing up. I did have clothing, but a good majority were
the remnants of clothing that was passed down to me.
Just as a starting place, I made an effort to see which of
those clothes I already had in my closet at least fit me the
way that I liked.

For about a week or two, I would take a selfie or
write down what I wore each day and how it made me feel
throughout the day. The clothes that didn't make me feel
comfortable, I thought about why and put in a pile to get
rid of. Did it feel too tight? Was it itchy? Maybe I just didn't
like how the clothes looked on my body. Sometimes I just
didn't like the color. Then, I did the same thing for the
clothes that DID make me feel good and that I wanted to

keep. I thought about why I liked it. Was it the color? Was it the texture of the fabric? Maybe I liked how it shaped my body and had gotten a few compliments on my outfit that day. When I collected enough data on my favorite fits, I started to go shopping for one or two other clothing items at a time that fit me in that same way. This was the first step into finding my style while on a budget.

Thankfully in todays world, most people have access to the areas listed in the Physiological Needs stage. Even if you have to have a live with someone else temporarily or get assistance from your local authorities to get these needs met. Take a look at how you operate within these physiological needs. Do you have any trauma traits that carried over from your childhood like I did with clothing, food, and shelter? If so, what can you do to address and correct those behaviors? Confronting this will create a strong foundation for your confidence to grow which is crucial to have in the fashion world.

Level two of Maslow's hierarchy is the Safety and Security Needs. These needs being met are what protects you from loosing your physiological needs back in the first level. This includes health, employment, property, and social ability. I personally like to add transportation here although it could be considered to be included in the property category. This stage was the most difficult for me because I struggled in every area here. As I mentioned before, my social skills already weren't the best growing up. Truth be told, our finances were in an even worse condition. Money felt so taboo in my household and if it was discussed, it would usually be in a tense argument with whatever bill collector company my mom was on the phone with. The lack of money literally effected everything else in life we experienced from childhood, all the way up into adulthood. This includes the unfashionable clothes I had. As a result, this greatly impacted my confidence for years. Now that I was an adult, it got to the point where I literally could not afford to be prideful or embarrassed about expressing my lack of knowledge in finances. I needed help and quick.

The reality is in this country, more money brings more options. More options bring more comfort and convenience. It also helps to be a bigger blessing to others. You cannot pour from an empty cup after all. This is where your employment and streams of income comes in handy. The money you earn from your job will be able to fund this transition from lack to comfort in order for you to secure your level of well-being. This is also the level where you can improve the needs you met in the physiological needs level. This is why getting your finances in order is so

important. This includes your spending plan (a.k.a.

budgeting), savings, credit, and investing. For me, I spent

a lot of time researching how people with money navigate

in life and made my own financial plans from there. What

did a comfortable life look like to me? How much time did I

want to spend working? What sort of things do I want to

be able to spend money on? I knew I didn't want to be

caught in the rat race of working just to pay bills, but I also

knew that not working at all would cut my sources of

income.

    In order to reach this stage, you may have to shift

your mindset around money. A lot of us were taught

through religion or our upbringing that money may be bad

or having a lot of it is greedy. I believe the opposite is true.

Having a healthy relationship with money in turn will allow

you to free your time doing what you find meaningful. It allows you to choose to move to a safer more resourceful environment instead of just the one you were born in. Maybe to get access to resources to protect yourself and your property. This also allows you to be able to afford a reliable vehicle to get you to and fro at your leisure. Having money also allows you to be able to buy more quality clothes that fit your style and personality, instead of only getting what can protect you from the weather like in the first level.

There is also something to be said about having much so that you can give back and pour into your family and community with the abundance. Think of how much good could come from being in the position to be able to help those in need. This also can effect the other area in the safety and security needs of improving your social ability. People are more willing to listen to someone who has the money to back up exactly what they speak on. Honestly, if I wasn't a seamstress and fashion designer, I would probably work in finances because I now understand just how much you can change a persons life by helping them excel with their finances. I even created my very own guide of how to keep and grow your money. Its called The 7 Walls of Wealth available on my website at www.aalichaw.com.

Another aspect of the safety and security needs is you have to be healthy. This means within both your body and your mind. Sadly, this is something most of Americans are known to struggle with across the globe. I am no expert in health, so it is best to consult with your doctor on your health needs. What I will say is, you know how you feel in your body. You probably also know exactly what to do about it if you are unhappy with what you see in the mirror. Confront it head on.

You can start small like I did. For me, I gain weight easily because I like to stress eat. Knowing this, I started small by first just being mindful of what I ate for a few weeks. Then, I would add small changes like a fruit smoothie to go with my breakfast or add just one salad a week to replace a meal. Later, I added walking to my routine. Just doing these things boosted my confidence, even if I didn't loose 20 pounds in a day. The inner knowing that I am addressing what I didn't like and following through on what I told myself I would do made a world of difference. The small changes were also easier to keep up with which as a result allowed me to look and feel better in my clothes.

As it relates to fashion, the safety and security needs level allows clothing to graduate from protecting you from basic hot and cold weather, to now functionality. For example, if you live in an area that is wet and rainy, you have the option of boots with the function of keeping you dry. This also includes a construction worker wearing a helmet and a reflector vest. It may not be very fashionable, but has the purpose to protect the worker from head injury and being clearly seen in dark places. This can even include having buttons, pockets, zippers or belt loops on your pants. Each detail has a function. For me, I know I spend a lot of time either sewing, running errands, or doing a light workout. That means the function of my clothing needed to match my daily lifestyle. This was the next step to shaping my style. By this time, I have a good sense of how I like my clothes to fit on me and what purpose I needed them for on a daily basis. Now I could start weeding out items from my closet that didn't meet these requirements.

Take a moment to reflect on if you feel a sense of safety and security within your life. Are you satisfied with the environment you live in? How about your way of getting around? Do you feel secure within your finances? Survey your closet and determine whether the function or purpose of the outfits you have match the needs your daily lifestyle calls for. If you notice that you have difficulty finding your style or you just don't like what you see in your closet, you might need to take a look at your current lifestyle. It's probably a good sign that you are in the middle of a personal shift. What you used to do before maybe is not want you want to do anymore. As my mom would say, "There's been a shift in the atmosphere."

At the middle of Maslow's pyramid, the third level is the Love and Belonging Needs. This is the point where you begin to crave some form of connection with another being. This includes friendships, pets, family, intimacy, and community. It may come as a surprise that this level was not listed as the first and starting place of the pyramid. Wouldn't family come first? Well, I agree that family is very important and has so many benefits to a person's life. However, what will you have to share with your family if you struggle with keeping food and shelter for yourself? Do you have the financial means to support your family? Is your health in a good condition to be able to protect and provide for your family? Without mastering the first two levels of your physiological and security needs, you may unintentionally be more harm than help to your family.

When you haven't successfully been able to take care of your own basic needs, it is more likely to become a heavy burden to those around you. It's like that saying we all know when you get on an airplane and the flight attendant says "In the event of an emergency, put your own face mask on first before you help others." Just think, if it was difficult for you to get these needs met for yourself, don't you think it will also be difficult for a family member who probably had a similar background and upbringing as you to do so too? How can a person meet the needs of two people when they barely can meet these needs for just one of themselves? Now think about if you were to put this adult burden on children. Unfortunately, this happens more common than not in my community. If an adult couldn't handle the load, how would it be fair to dump the issue on a child who knows less and has less than a full grown adult? Personally. I think this behavior coming from an adult is neglectful at best, and child abuse

at its worst. Get your own physiological and security needs

met first before having a family or taking care of family

burdens. This way, you have a lot more to share with your

family and lessen the likely hood of an estranged and

traumatic relationship with a loved one.

For me, when I was in the middle of what I called

my quarter-life crisis, I believe this stage of the pyramid

was the reason why. I was stepping into adulthood and

had no community. Both my parents were in two different

states, I was away from most of my family, the friends and

resources I made before, and I didn't know hardly anyone

in this new community I was dropped in. It was time I

started making some connections. I started first with small

conversations with my parents on the phone. Asking my

mom about what her life looked like when she was my age

and asking my dad about how he wanted to name me after the 90's R&B singer Aaliyah when I was born. Then deeper conversations surfaced. We began discussing childhood traumas, both mine and theirs. Getting to know my parents and lineage on a deeper level fueled my sense of belonging in teaching me where I came from. I felt less lonely in the world. I also learned that my grandmothers on both sides were also seamstresses before they passed. I had been carrying on a legacy and had no idea!

I then stared to take trips to back home to Ohio and Georgia to visit my family who I'd missed so much. Then, I took trips to Texas, New York and Florida where I didn't know anyone just to explore. Without even realizing it, this was the first time I had been successfully operating in three levels of the pyramid at the same time. I was handling my basic needs at home, was learning to be more financially secure, I could get the type of food and clothing that I actually wanted, I kept my health in mind, and now started traveling to building strong connections with my family. The adventures forced me to come out of my shy and anxiety filled behaviors to interact with strangers. Whether it was TSA at the airport, the cashier at a store, or the receptionist at the front desk in the hotel lobby. This also helped me to speak up for myself.

I was now learning to practice being assertive with my wants and needs. Because most companies dealing with travel are geared to focus on customer service, it made being assertive feel less confrontational. It was a huge shift for me since I could never do things like this when I was younger. However, because traveling was never a priority growing up, it almost felt wasteful of my hard earned money. Again, I would remind myself that I added it to the budget to fulfill my mission of connection. Now that I could afford more things, it helped me to learn how to spend money guilt free. I would even congratulate myself along the way because it felt like in doing these small things, I was breaking generational curses. After a while, I finally began to view travel as an investment into myself.

In fashion, sharing trends and styles can also create a sense of belonging and create social connections within communities. For example at certain events, ceremonies, and celebrations, there are certain cloths and styles that groups of people wear which represents a piece of their identity and even their heritage. This is true for all kinds of cultures and races such as African, Asian, and Hispanic for example. This can even be something as simple as if you are a member at a gym, you dress in gym attire when you go to workout. This alone can create a sense of belonging

because everyone is dressed for the same shared

purpose. This knowledge is even used in the workforce at

jobs. Why do you think most companies have a uniform or

dress code standard? This is to ensure everyone

understands and shares the same purpose of the

company. This is also to represent the company brand as a

unit.

At the fourth level of Maslow's hierarchy, second

from the top is Esteem. This includes respect, self-esteem,

status, recognition, strength, confidence, achievement,

and the need to be a unique individual. This is that full

circle moment I was talking about earlier. These are all

areas that have the greatest impact on your fashion sense.

I love using Maslow's pyramid because when looking at

the hierarchy of needs, it begins to unravel why it can be

so difficult for many to have self-esteem and confidence.
Do you see how there are three whole stages that come
before achieving esteem that need to be addressed before
you even begin to walk into your confidence? And because
these stages are also interconnected, if you struggle to
maintain one stage, it is highly likely that you also struggle
in one or more of the other the stages. Each builds upon
the other as a foundation. If the foundation is weak, it
won't be strong enough to support the others. As a result,
you may end up feeling lost, anxious, lonely, depressed,
and feeling low self-worth. This explains why I felt that I
was in a quarter life crisis before the age of 25. I hadn't
done any intentional work to build my foundation. As a
result, I was unable to reach the final stage at the top of
Maslow's pyramid. Because the final stage is the most
powerful and less common to master, I'll revisit this to go
more into depth in the final chapter.

So how exactly do you build esteem? Again I looked towards Google. Some of the results that popped up included affirmations, setting goals, seeking feedback, and power posing in the mirror. Well to put it bluntly, the affirmations felt fake, I set huge goals then beat myself up when I didn't reach them, I felt I had gotten enough feedback still slightly scarred by the experience I had back with the shop owner, and the only power pose I could think of was standing at a military's attention stance in the mirror, which just felt awkward and didn't match my personality. Clearly I needed to adjust a few things.

I started with affirmations. "I am confident, " I repeated to myself. Although I was saying the words out loud, deep down I knew I didn't fully believe it. No matter how many times I repeated it, I knew it wasn't quite true.

Believing that one day I would just wake up on top of the

world with all the confidence in the world felt far fetched.

So, I tweaked the words to what felt more realistic and

believable to me. "I am learning to be confident." "Every

day my confidence can grow." This felt a lot more genuine

because instead of falsely proclaiming that I was

something I knew I wasn't, I phrased it to reflect a

progressional change. It was far easier for me to believe

this way.

I also began to set small goals for myself. First, I

would task myself to get small things done that I knew I

had put off. For example, I would get gas the night before

rather than saying "I'll just do it in the morning." I've

actually never shared this with anyone before now, but

when I got to the gas station, I would only get gas at pump

number one. It may sound silly, but I was subconsciously

telling myself that I was number one to build my self

esteem. Being shy and always afraid to be first of anything,

this helped me to visualize what being first looked like.

Even if it was only to get gas. I also started to food prep for

myself knowing that I get hungry around certain times so

instead of snacking or going to a drive thru, my food was

already prepared. Then, once I proved to myself that I can

get things done quicker than I thought before, I gave

myself larger tasks.

I started to add into my budget some small

privileges I could enjoy. For example, I would book hair

and nail appointments. This may be small for someone

else, but for me spending money on hair and nails regularly

weren't things I was used to because they weren't a

priority for us growing up. At first, I felt guilty for spending money on what I used to feel to be vain expenses before I addressed my security needs level. I simply to reminded myself that I deserved to look nice. "I'm worth it," I would tell myself. I was learning to give myself self care. I also had to forgive myself for not doing things like this sooner. I knew I wasn't taught things like self care and finances when I was younger, so of course it would feel foreign at first.

I also dedicated myself to becoming a forever student. I began reading books back to back. Self help books, business books, psychology books, and books on relationships were all interesting to me. I was obsessed. I wanted to learn more and gain as much knowledge as I could because honestly, I felt I was already behind for my age. Amazon's Audible is still my personal favorite for books while on the go.

I even took classes for business, finances and sewing. Studying deeper into my craft allowed me to focus on a personal strength I had. I increased my skills, which in turn allowed me to increase my prices for my sewing orders. This simultaneously strengthened my security and safety needs. The more I learned, the better I got with practice and the more valuable I felt. It was then that I started to keep a journal. I would write what I learned that day, how I felt about it, and how I planned to implement it into my life. Often times, I would share what I learned with my mom or Morgan or whoever would listen in hopes that I would bring some sort of value to their lives or businesses too.

Getting more involved in local events helped with both my sense of belonging and my esteem. Going to the holiday festivities at the local park, always wearing something I sewed myself, allowed me to see what my community actually looked like. I got many compliments on what I made to wear and even had strangers want to take pictures with me. Because I had gotten involved in my community, I started to get recognized more often. My picture even ended up being featured on the NAACP social media page one year at the local Juneteenth Festival. I also started getting invited to the homecoming fashion show at HBCUs like Livingstone College and Johnson C. Smith University. Then, I began branching off to fashion shows at High Point Fashion Week and doing community work there too.

These were environments that celebrated and appreciated both me and my craft. I didn't stop there either. I made sure to get involved in groups and classes where we all had the same goal in mind. I went to yoga

class with my amazing instructor Janet, where we all were

there for health. That meant I automatically belonged

simply because I wanted to improve my health too.

Being in yoga also helped me to get comfortable with my

body. There are many positions and stances in yoga that

are considered power poses, but felt less awkward than

the military pose I tried before in the mirror. In yoga class, I

didn't think of them as power poses, but just as stretching.

I always love when Janet would end the class saying,

"Thank you so much for taking time for yourself. I hope

whatever it was you came for, you received. Safe trips

home and remember it's more important to have the time,

than to wear the watch." These classes boosted my

confidence, improved my overall health, and allowed me to

meet even more amazing people from my community.

I also drove to Greensboro, NC to attend a high heels dance class. Coming from a shy and very Christian background, this was way out of my comfort zone! I felt I needed to really challenge myself to break me out of my shell even more. Before I started my confidence journey, I gained weight. Frankly, I was the heaviest I had ever been. I now had extra curves that I didn't know what to do with. I was out of tune with my body. While yoga was a fun and gentle beginning for my self improvement journey, it didn't push me completely out of my comfort zone like I knew I needed.

The high heels class required you come face to face with yourself in the mirror. Your every move is visible from head to toe. It was extremely confrontational. At the beginning of each class, the instructor Deanna would always ask you to share something you felt was iconic about yourself. We would do warmups in the mirror and every single girl in the room encouraged each other. There were no such thing as mistakes, only freestyles. I knew right away that this class was exactly what I needed. My mom of course expressed her clear disapproval for the "inappropriate" class when she found out about it, but I knew I was operating on a higher purpose. I was finding myself. I was realigning.

I also started looking for other opportunities to give and be of service. I went back into my closet and started going through all the items I couldn't fit or didn't want anymore and either tossed or donated them. I knew somewhere out there somebody might be in a similar situation that I was in when I was younger and maybe could only afford second hand clothes. Now I knew I could bring value to strangers that I probably would never even meet. To this day, I clean out my closet every year and donate to Goodwill or find one of those clothing donation stands in parking lots.

Although these may sound like small things, psychologically I was training myself to get used to taking up space, being present, and making my own mark in the world. At the same time, I also built an entire community of people who encourage, support, and teach me new information. I built my own foundation of people I could rely on in different areas of my life. To this day, this is a priceless asset to me and my journey of life and my community keeps growing even larger.

This esteem level in the pyramid also is the point where your creativity and self expression begin to awaken, which is where the core of fashion branches from. Fashion plays a significant role in building self esteem and confidence by allowing people to express their personality freely. Wearing clothes that reflect your creativity and uniqueness can boost your esteem especially when you receive complements from others. This positive validation from others encourages you to want to continue operating in your creativity and express your full personality on a regular basis.

These first four levels in Maslow's Hierarchy of Needs are what the mental fitting room allows you to test and try out. Reflect on what each these levels look like for you in your life. Once you've started the internal work and addressing these areas, your true sense of style will begin to unravel. You would have effectively caused a domino effect. While I was slowly shaping my new lifestyle one level at a time, the changes had rippled into my clothing style. What I thought about myself, the places I went to, and activities I was now involved in called for a different look than what I originally had in my closet. I could visibly see how most outfits no longer matched the feel or the purpose of the new lifestyle I had created.

I believe conquering all these areas is necessary for you to discover your style, afford the clothes you like, and feel good in your garments from the inside out. To aid you in your journey, I've created a list of books, mentors, and many more resources that were helpful to me in these multiple areas of my life. You can find these resources listed on my website at www.aalichaw.com. Now, it's time to get ready to take your closet to the next level!

The 5 Body Shapes

Okay, now we're getting to the fun part! Go ahead and celebrate yourself because you have put in so much work to get this far! It is not easy to look at yourself in the mirror to not only identify your shortcomings, but address them too. Everywhere you go, you bring yourself with you. That's why it's important to get to know who you are and how you impact the spaces around you. No matter who you are, where you live, or what you believe in, being self aware is first step in nurturing your confidence and self worth. It is the only way to bring health, wealth, happiness, and wholeness into your life. Self awareness is so important because it is not only included in so many aspects of a successful life, but also fuels your confidence. The goal of the practices discussed in the previous chapter from Maslow's pyramid is to begin bringing awareness to yourself and your unique lifestyle. When you thoroughly know yourself, you can accurately dress yourself.

Once you've tapped into your overall lifestyle, you may begin to discover that you lean more towards certain looks or images that match your personality. Your image is any message or feeling you want to portray to those around you, about you. Think about how you want other people to view you when they see you. Although it is a little unfair, people do judge you based off of their first impression of you. Remember, energy responds to energy. Don't take this to heart or feel too deeply about it though.

Without a proper sit down conversation with you and paying full attention to you over periods of time, it is impossible for a person to really get to know who you are. And quite frankly, we don't exactly have enough time or may not even desire for every stranger we come across to have long deep conversations with us. However, this quick snapshot of your appearance can be used to your advantage. The best part about your image is that it can also be changed as often as you want it to depending on what you feel the need is in that environment.

For example, let's say after reading the Fitting Room chapter, you decided to start the new habit of working out first thing in the morning, before you're awake enough to talk yourself out of it. You then proceed to put on your workout clothes and running shoes and head to the gym or walk around your neighborhood. To the strangers who may see you working out, your image to them is that you are

athletic and care deeply about your health. They have no

idea that you just started to do this for the first time that

day. And you probably aren't going to tell everyone you

lock eyes with that this is your first time either! After

awhile, working out becomes a habit and a part of your

new lifestyle. This then calls for your wardrobe to keep up

with this lifestyle. This leads to a more intentional wardrobe

which as a result will fuel your confidence. Do you see how

it's all connected?

I find that when you have a closet that reflects the

areas you've mastered in Maslow's pyramid, you are more

satisfied with what you wear. That means that your closet

is well rounded with a different variety of clothing that

protects you from the cold weather, clothes that allow your

skin to breathe and cool off in the hot weather, clothes that are functional to your everyday needs or for your working environment, clothes that represent the different groups and clubs you are a part of and clothes that show off your unique personality through different color combinations. A good way to learn what your style may be is to take a selfie of yourself everyday for about two weeks. Document your mood, what you liked, disliked, and any compliments you may have gotten about each outfit of the day. You can document this in a journal or make a quick video for yourself on your phone. Another area to take a look at is the places that you visit frequently. Where are you majority of the time? Do you spend a lot of your time at work or maybe the gym? The goal is if you spend majority of your time at work, it wouldn't make much sense to wear or have a lot of club type outfits in your closet. Similarly, if you know you're more on the athletic side and spend a lot of time at the gym and outdoors in shorts or leggings, you may not be interested in having too many dainty dresses in the closet.

Another way to learn your style is to think about what celebrities you pay attention to the most. What is their style? How do they dress? It's likely that your personality can relate to theirs in some way and you may want to mimic what they wear to find inspiration. They don't have to have your exact body shape, as we can tailor the look specifically to you and your body shape. Remember it's okay to have a nice mix of different styles to match your different environments and moods. And you can always decide if these styles need to change again over time.

My recent celebrity favorites are Fantasia, Zendaya, Kelly Rowland, and Teyana Taylor. I love to feel as feminine as possible when going on a night out or fashion events so dresses like the ones they wear are always a go to for me. With my new lifestyle, the places I frequent like my fashion shows, have a dress code leaning towards the formal or dressy side. I do love to get my workout time in too, so I keep a light collection of yoga and walking clothes. When I'm not going out or exercising, it is an absolute must that I feel comfortable at my sewing office or at home.

For me, I like to base my image on the location and the occasion of what I'm going to. I think about where I will be so I can determine if it will be appropriate to wear business or casual attire and also get an idea of what the weather or temperature will be like. You can decide this by simply Googling the location you are going to and try to find pictures if you can. Then, I consider the purpose and theme and try to match that. For example, a kids birthday party at an indoor bounce house would call for a different outfit than an adult birthday party at a rooftop restaurant and bar. Your image always works best when you match the theme or purpose of the event, then throw in a sprinkle of your personality with different colors and textures in fabric. This is when you start to hear the phrase that someone "understood the assignment" when seeing their outfit.

When it comes to body shapes, there are five main categories. These categories focus on the measurements mainly of your chest and shoulders, your waist, and your hips. It's best to get yourself measured, but you can just look at yourself in the mirror to determine which category you fall into. The categories are Hourglass, Rectangle, Inverted Triangle, Pear, and Apple. Each of these shapes have male versions, so the same basic principles apply. In my viral video on social media, I broke down how Issa Rae wore a beautiful two piece outfit to the Beyoncé World Tour Concert and why this fit worked perfectly for her. As I go in depth for all five categories here, I want to remind you not to get too carried away with the names of each category or your exact measurement numbers.

All body shapes can be dressed well. And it's entirely possible to transition from one category to another, then back again. We are all spiritual beings just having a human experience. That means our bodies have been constantly changing ever since we were inside our mother's womb. You wouldn't beat yourself up about how you don't fit into your newborn onesie anymore would you? Give yourself grace and space. It's all a journey remember? Also, these suggestions are to be viewed at as just that, a suggestion. These are a guide not laws, rules, or regulations. Use what you like, and feel free to leave the rest. This is your journey and your style so there are no wrong answers. I also created a printable diagram that illustrates displays the different body types shapes. you can find this on my website at www.aalichaw.com.

The most well-known And highly celebrated body shape is by no surprise the **Hourglass** body type. The hourglass shape means that the measurement around your chest and hips are relatively equal in width, give or take a few inches, while your waist measurement is well defined and noticeably smaller than both. This body shape is the most celebrated because it's what the human eye finds the most balanced. Just think about what the human skeleton looks like. Both the ribs and the hips are often wide, while the only bone positioned in between those two is the spine. It then starts to make sense that we feel this hourglass shape is the most natural. We like to see balance and the hourglass body shape is the most visually proportionate. So much so, the other four body shapes are dressed to give the illusion of mimicking this body shape. Celebrities such as Fantasia, Megan thee Stallion, Jennifer Lopez, and Scarlett Johansson all have the hourglass figure.

When styling the hourglass figure, there are many options to play around with. Because this figure is the most proportionate, it can easily be the most versatile when it comes to styling. Your main area of focus would always be to emphasize your waist. Fitted and tailored clothing is ideal. When shopping or reviewing your existing wardrobe, you want to focus on clothing that hugs the body, but not too tight or restrictive.

If you're wearing a dress, have the waist area tailored in for more of a snug fit. You can also add a cute thin belt to the waist. Tops with a V-neck line flatter the shape well while still following the natural silhouette of the body. When wearing jeans or pants, try a fitted or straight leg. You may have to opt for a larger size that fits your hips, but be sure to have the waist tailored in or wear a belt. The same goes for wearing any kind of two-piece outfit or a jumpsuit. You want to keep the balance of proportions so that the overall look is harmonious. Pencil skirts, wrap dresses, and peplum tops all follow the body's natural shape and highlights your curves. Leggings and high waisted skinny jeans are also flattering.

Stretchy fabrics are your best friend to complement your curves. You'll also want to invest in supportive undergarments. When accessorizing, again you want to draw attention to the waist by wearing belts or with a nice statement handbag. While solid colors work the absolute best for this shape, don't be afraid to play around with print and patterns. Vertical stripes, color blocking, and textured fabrics all are fun ways to enhance the hourglass figure. Your waist is your strongest point so build your outfit with it as the main focus.

For the fellas, I didn't forget about you guys! The male version of this shape is called the **Trapezoid**. The chest measurement is relatively equal to the hips, while the waist is defined and smaller than both. Celebrities such as Micheal B. Jordan, Dwayne "The Rock" Johnson, and Ryan Reynolds fit into this category. Guys want to emphasize on your broad shoulders as well as the tailored in waist. Shirts and jackets should be fitted and tapered at the waist. Pants and shorts should be tapered in to follow the natural silhouette of the thigh to calf to ankle, but not too tight. If you like patterns, they should go vertically down the body. You want to avoid access bulk in fits and go for darker colored tops. When accessorizing, you want to draw attention to your face or waist. This can be achieved with scarves, necklaces, or belts.

Next, we have the **Rectangle** body type. This may also be referred to as square or straight but is referred to as the same name for both men and women. This body shape means that all three of your measurements for chest, waist, and hips are relatively the same width straight down. A few celebrities that fit into this category are Issa Rae, Zendaya, Jada Pinkett Smith and Coi Leray.

For the rectangle figure, you want to really define the waist. Any dresses, shirts, or pants should be tailored to the waist. Two piece outfits work really well to disrupt the "boxy" silhouette. When shopping or reviewing your own closet, any top that draws attention to the chest is a must. Go for tops that elongate the neckline and draw the eye upwards such as deep V-necks, scoop-necks, off shoulder, and sweetheart necklines. Structured tops and jackets with elaborate detailing or extra padding in the shoulders are a go to. Similarly, with bottoms and skirts that have elaborate detailing or structured shapes that give the illusion of hips are great to play around with.

Sweaters or jackets should have either large puffy sleeves, or fitted to the arm with extra padding at the shoulders. Slightly baggy clothing can be fun to play around with whether a puffy dress, baggy jeans or oversized jackets. If wearing a skirt, look for circle or maxi skirts with plenty of movement and volume around the hips. With a fitted pencil skirt or dress, try one that goes just above the knee or down to the ankles. Preferably an attention grabbing color or heavy textured fabric. This draws the attention of the eye down the leg adding more dimension to the outfit. The same works with baggy, flare, or wide legged pants. You also want to play with lots of patterned fabrics! Remember, we want to bring more attention to the chest, shoulders and hip areas.

Male celebrities that have the rectangle body shape are Daniel Kaluuya, Chris Brown, Jason Statham, and Stephen Curry. The goal when dressing in this category is to draw attention towards your face or lower half. Guys with the rectangle body shape should wear clothing that emphasizes broad shoulders such as jackets or blazers with extra padding in the shoulders and neck lines that include V-neck and scoop neck. Tops should be tailored in at the waist and maybe add some layering such as a scarf or statement tie to add dimension. Pants and shorts should follow the natural line of the leg to allow movement.

Then we have the **Inverted Triangle** body shape. This body shape features your chest on the bustier side or shoulders very broad measuring to be your widest, then your waist slightly smaller, then your hips as the narrowest part of the three. Celebrities such as Simone Biles, Sherri Shepherd, Naomi Campbell, and Wendy Williams fit into this category.

The key to dressing this body shape is to highlight the lower half of the body. When shopping or reviewing your closet, avoid leggings and pencil skirts. You want to give the illusion of curves by defining your waist, and creating volume from the hips down. Wide leg pants, maxi skirts, and circle skirts can achieve this. You can also create the illusion of curves by wearing long skirts or pants with slits down the leg or elaborate detailing. Don't be afraid to play around with different textures in fabric and bright colors on the lower half of your body.

Moderate V-neck or unique asymmetrical tops work really well. Wrap dresses and peplum tops aid in bringing balance to your outfits. Stick with neutral or darker colors for your upper half. Short sleeve tops should be fitted around the shoulders to avoid adding extra volume. However, long sleeve tops should have some movement or flare to them as they add volume to your middle and lower half. Tops should also flare out just below the waistline. It may also help to add layering. Cardigans and structure jackets can add balance to your upper and lower halves.

Male celebrities that fit into the inverted triangle category are Usain Bolt, Vin Diesel and John Cena. Men also want to draw attention to emphasize their lower half. Tops and jackets for guys should be fitted to the shoulders and chest while having a slight flare at the hips. Instead of high collared shirts that draw attention back up to your broad shoulders, go for V-neck shirts. Short sleeve shirts should have a fitted sleeve while long sleeves should be fitted at the shoulder, but loose or flowing at the wrist. Straight leg pants or cargo pants are a go to and you should avoid any skinny jeans or tight fitting shorts or pants. Layering cardigans and jackets will help balance your top and lower halves.

Now we have the **Pear** Body shape. The measurements for this shape are where your shoulders are fairly narrow or a smaller bust. Your waist may be slightly wider than your chest, resulting in your hips being the widest measurement. Coco Jones, Chloe Bailey, Priyanka Chopra, and Janelle Monet are all celebrities who fit into this body shape.

When dressing the pear body shape, you want to draw attention to your upper half. Add dimension to the chest and shoulder areas by choosing tops with elaborate details, patterns, and textures. Play around with bold prints in fabric and bright colors for tops to create visual balance. Statement pieces such as scarves, elaborate earrings and necklaces keep the attention upward.

When shopping or reviewing your closet, you want to have clothes that are tailored at the waist. Look for A-line skirts where it begins fitted to the waist then gradually flares out at the bottom hem. Mermaid skirts are a great option too. Dark colored bottoms work well to balance this shape. For pants, boot cut or flare are a good option to smooth out the silhouette line from the waist to the ankle. Choosing structured fabrics such as denim, cotton, and twill create a clean and supportive feel.

The male version of this shape is called the **Triangle.** The shoulders and chest are narrow compared to the hips and waist. Some celebrity examples include Chris Rock, Samuel L Jackson, and Robert Downey Jr. Guys want to draw attention to the upper body. You want to add volume to the shoulder areas. Jackets and blazers should have extra padding in the shoulders and fitted at the waist. V- necklines and scoop neck shirts that elongate the neck line work well. Play with patterns and extra detailing with tops to draw the eye upwards. Look for darker color bottoms and avoid excessive baggy pants like cargos. A straight leg can help balance the overall look.

And finally we have the **Apple** body shape. The features of the apple body shape measures your waist being the widest and fullest part of your body. While your chest may be equal or slightly smaller than the midsection, your hips often measure as the narrowest of the three. Celebrities such as Queen Latifa, Lizzo, Da'vine Joy Randolph, and Melissa McCarthy fit into this category.

When shopping or reviewing your closet with the apple body shape, you want to opt for clothing that draws attention away from the midsection and towards your bust and legs. You can enhance the bust and leg areas by creating the illusion of a defined waistline. You can achieve this by forming a waistline line in the space starting right below the bust, and just above the belly. Go for clothing that is tailored in at this area. V-neck and scoop neck tops elongate the neckline and draws attention upwards.

Wrap dresses work really well because they wrap exactly in that space between the bust and belly and gently skim over the midsection without bunching. Flowing fabrics are your friend for tops and bottoms to allow movement and comfort. Lean towards skirts and pants that elongate the legs and play around with different lengths. Lengths that hit right at or slightly above the knee are flattering for this shape. Patterns that run vertically are great for skirts and pants and darker shade colors work best. Accessories such as statement necklaces, earrings and handbags help to balance the overall look.

The male version of this body shape is the **Oval**. Men with an oval body shape are featured as having rounded bellies with the midsection being the widest measurement compared to the chest and hips. Celebrities that have this body shape include Ice Cube, Cedric the Entertainer, and Jack Black. Guys want to choose styles that elongate the torso and draw the eye upwards. You want to go for shirts with scoop, necks and slight V-necks. Vertical seams in shirts and vertical stripes and patterns help to achieve this elongated appearance. Shirts and suit jackets should be tailored in slightly at the space just below your chest and just above your belly this creates a more defined waist

It may be tempting to wear baggy clothing, but this should be avoided as it does not give your body a defined looking shape. Tailored clothing is a must have for tops and bottoms. Lean towards darker shades in clothing. Consider taking advantage of layering, such as pairing a fitted T-shirt with a jacket or cardigan. When accessorizing, you want to draw attention upwards towards the face with ties or scarves for example.

In the fashion industry, the most desired body shape for the red carpet and in fashion shows is on the thinner side with minimal curves. Although this may seem a bit shallow, there is a reason behind this. Making gowns in this industry is often very expensive and it requires an awful lot of hours in labor to piece together. If you are dressing a model on the smaller side, this means you will need less fabric and materials than a person that has more body surface to cover. Less fabric means less cost in materials. When drawing out each pattern piece of what will be sewing together to make a garment, those on the thinner side often fit perfectly in a pre-made pattern piece and will need far less adjustments made to their garment versus someone curvier. This smaller size also makes shipping cost cheaper and needed materials more likely to arrive in a timely manner from other countries when ordering quality materials. This is crucial when in a fast paced industry, especially if you are dressing more than one person for a red carpet event or fashion show. In addition, the designer of these high-end brands rarely ever make their own pieces themselves after designing them. They always have a team of seamstresses and tailors that actually do the cutting, stitching, sewing, and beading. Each of these jobs takes an excruciating amount of time and meticulous coordination. That's why the finished product is so expensive if the brand decides to actually sell the piece.

Unfortunately, this causes high-end brands to have little knowledge in how to properly dress those on a larger scale than the thin standard. Due to being more expensive and time consuming, these brands may not even be willing to take on creating a garment for someone of a larger size. This is when I like to look for brands and designers who aren't afraid of breaking away from traditional models. In 2016, comedian and actress Leslie Jones made it publicly known that for the premier of her first big role in the Hollywood movie *Ghostbusters,* she had so much difficulty finding a designer to dress her. She was refused over and over by well known brands. Designer Christian Siriano then took it upon himself to take on the mission of creating a gown for her which ended up being the highlight of the premier.

Because my brand is rooted in building confidence for women of all sizes, I strive to included as many shapes of woman I can when styling and creating. I have the honor of doing this every time I am invited to be a part of a fashion show. I hand select my models and make it my business to find women that are different shapes, sizes, and skin tones within my collection. While the models that choose to participate are sometimes out of my control, I still like to encourage everyone to come to tryouts and rehearsals. I believe it is so important to have accurate representation of how beauty comes in all different forms. This is also a fun way for me as a designer to challenge my skills when designing and creating. After all I feel that you can't truly call yourself a real designer if you only have knowledge on just one body shape.

Shapeshifting

Now that we have covered the five main body types and how to style them, I know that there are still some parts of our body you may need a little more time adjusting to if you are in the process of transitioning between shapes. While your confidence level is growing over time, you still might feel uncomfortable about certain areas on your body. That's okay! When styling and getting dressed, we all have target areas on our bodies that we either want to enhance or draw attention away from. Because these areas are not always included or focused on in the overall body shapes, we'll review some of the most common areas of attention separately. These target area hacks can be combined with your suggested body shape hacks to create the ultimate shape shift. This is also a great opportunity to add in more of your personality for styling.

1.) The Stomach

Contrary to what most may think, having a round belly is not reserved for only those with an oval or apple body shape. You can have an hourglass figure, and still have a round belly. The only difference is that the width of your chest and hips in the hourglass figure are originally still wider than your stomach, so you still fall in the same category. If you want to enhance your stomach area, say for a pregnancy photoshoot, two piece outfits are the go to. Any dress with a cut out section in the midsection will work to show off the stomach. Any fitted dress or skirt can draw attention to the midsection. If the goal is to disguise the stomach, you want to go with flowing fabrics that just skim over the stomach and end just below the hip line. Wrap dresses, high waisted pants, or shorts where the waistline is in the space just below the bust and just above the stomach work well too. Circle skirts, dresses or skirts that are gathered to one side to create a folded silhouette also help to mask the midsection.

2.) The Booty

Let's face it. People these days like butts. If you were born curvy and want to enhance the booty, any stretch material will work. Workout pants, like leggings or yoga stretch pants always do the trick. The leggings with color block sections are very popular currently. The area covering the booty is usually a lighter shade than the rest of the leg and more often have a scrunched detailing in the back center.

Any kind of bright colors such as white, tan, and light gray also draws attention to this area. If you aren't as curvy and want to give the illusion of a booty, peplum tops, circle skirts and wide leg or baggy pants can achieve this. If you have curves and want to conceal them, possibly for work purposes, go for long flowing skirts or straight legged pants. Preferably in black, navy, or dark gray colors due to dark colors having a slimming effect to the eye. A shirt or jacket that flows loosely just below the hip line will also aid in concealing the hips.

3.) The Chest

To enhance the chest area, tops such as deep V-neck and scoop necks are the first pick. Off shoulder tops and spaghetti strap tops may also achieve this. Wearing stripes horizontally has a widening effect to the eye, so tops with a horizontal pattern will widen the look of your bust.

Surprisingly, turtlenecks help to accentuate the bust as well. Bright colored tops, such as yellow, red and pink aso bring attention to the chest area. Try accessorizing with elaborate jewelry, such as a Cuban link, dangle necklaces, and dangling earrings to draw the eye up to the chest. For those who are extremely busty and want to disguise that area, a moderate, V-neck can get the job done. It may sound counterintuitive, but wearing a turtleneck, for example, actually causes the bust to look bigger. The silhouette of a turtleneck begins at the neck, which is thin in comparison to your chest and shoulders which is wide. This causes a drastic contrast with your wide bust and results in making it look wider. A moderate V-neck disrupts this wide contrast between the neck, shoulders and chest. Asymmetrical tops have the same effect and are a great option to distract from having a large bust. Dark colored fabrics help to slim the area too so look for black, navy, dark gray, and brown colors.

4.) The Legs

If you want to enhance your legs, shorts, mini skirts, and dresses with a high slit are perfect for a leg moment. High waisted bottoms with brighter colors also draw the eye down. To elongate the leg giving the illusion of being taller, of course heels are a go-to. Open toe sandals or low top sneakers with can do this as well. Pattern designs that are small in scale and run vertically works well. Guys want to opt for pointed toe shoes that are the same color as their pants to add the illusion of height. Pants that end just pass your ankles, can also elongate the leg. Solid colors in bottoms can also be used to elongate the legs. To disguise the legs, baggy or wide leg pants will do the job. Long flowing skirts will help to conceal the legs too. If you are tall and looking to appear shorter, break up the look of the

leg with color block pants or ripped jeans. Play around

with horizontal patterns in bottoms. Wearing thigh high

boots, or heels that come up the leg will help in disrupting

the look of lengthy legs. The same works for high top

sneakers, maybe even with high socks.

5.) The Arms

To enhance the arms, any top that has little to no coverage

on the arms is best. Sleeves such as cap sleeves, halter

tops, and spaghetti straps also show off the arms and

shoulders. Of course sleeveless tops are best to achieve

this. Fitted or tailored sleeves can also help enhance your

muscles. To minimize or shrink the look of your arms, play

around with longer length in sleeves. Fabric choice is also

something to pay attention to. Thicker fabrics can add bulk

to arms on the thinner side. In contrast, light and flowing

fabrics can help conceal arms larger in size. Elaborate

details on the shoulders and chest areas can also draw the

attention away from the arms.

Because we are all human I understand that

sometimes even after doing all this, you may still be

unhappy with the way you look in the mirror. If you've been

consistently in the gym, making changes in your diet,

picking clothes that flatter your existing shape and

dressing your target areas accordingly, there is also the

option of shape wear. I don't like to start off recommending

shape wear right away because I feel it only masks your

unliked areas without embracing them first. It's like treating

the symptoms but never addressing the cause. Although

easy and more convenient, it doesn't really build lasting

confidence in loving the body you currently have. It could

also end up making you feel even more uncomfortable and restricted throughout the day.

Finally as a last resort, and preferably only if you have diagnosed medical conditions that limit your diet or physical activity AND if your doctor approves you for it, there are doctors all across the US that can alter any part of your body you like. Again I don't like to start off with this type of solution for fixing a bodily problem you are unhappy with. I strongly believe that working from the inside out verses the outside in is more effective in the long run and satisfying. I know that if you put in the hard work to make a change in your life, you are less likely to revert back to how you were before because of all you had to go through. It also builds so much trust in yourself because you take pride in knowing you are to thank for bettering yourself. It's like when you did all the hard work to get a room clean and the moment you finish, you just step back

and observe the great job you did. You are also likely to

keep that room clean longer verses if you just had

someone else to do it for you. However, I also can't deny

that we live in a time where convenience runs our world. If

you feel this is your only option, make sure you consult

with your doctors to ensure that any procedure you get

won't compromise your health. Be sure you DO YOUR

RESEARCH beforehand!!

Color Coordination

My favorite part of an outfit is to look for an overall coordination. Nothing is more haunting to me than to see an outfit have a missed opportunity to be great because of an uncoordinated look. This could mean the colors are off, the fabric textures don't mix well, or one portion of the outfit competes with another giving an unbalanced feel. This can result in the overall outfit looking thrown together last minute, unflattering to the body shape, or even putting the person wearing the outfit in a visible unpleasant mood.

My strongest point as a fashion designer is my distinct eye for color. At my latest fashion show at High Point Fashion Week in North Carolina, one of the most repeated compliments I got was the collection's color spectrum. I got the same feedback at the fashion show I was featured in the year prior. When it comes to color shades, I like to group colors that complement each other. Both the color and texture of a fabric you choose for an outfit is an opportunity to express your personality and individuality. There are three ways I feel colors can be complementary to each other:

- Colors are in the same color family such as pink, red, and purple
- One color or pattern is paired with a neutral color such as black, white, grey, or tan

- A color is paired with its opposite such as red and green, orange and blue, and yellow and purple.

If you are first starting out in fashion, my rule of thumb is usually no more than three colors present in an entire outfit. This doesn't exactly have to include jewelry, belts, handbags, and shoes, but no more than three colors total if you can. Associating colors with each other in an outfit usually consist of two main colors and one accent color or pattern. This holy trinity is supported by the suggested rule of 60/30/10. This rule suggest that you build an outfit with one color as the dominant throughout the outfit. This one color will be present in about 60% of the overall look. The 30% color is a color that complements the dominant. This color should not over shadow or upstage the dominant color. And finally the 10% accent. The 10% accent color can be any wildcard or pattern that still supports both the dominant and complementing colors. Because the accent color is usually the most eye-catching if it is alone and upstage the dominant color, we would only allow 10% of the overall look to consist of this color or pattern. This rule can also be applied with different fabric textures.

For example, say you have a fitted red dress on and paired it with a classic pair of all black heels. You might even put on black accessories like black dangle earrings, hat, and a black watch. Then you grab a handbag with a fierce, leopard print. The color red would be your dominant color of 60%, the shoes, hat and jewelry would be your supporting color of 30% and the leopard handbag would be the 10%. Now there are some fabrics that have patterns which include more than three colors and that's okay. What I like to do in this instance is allow that one

multi-color piece to take up the majority of your outfit.
Then for your accessories, pick a color within the multi-
color piece that isn't as noticeable. That color is what your
accessories should be.

Each color also stimulates a mood within the wearer
and those around that see them. Colors are known to have
certain individual meanings to them. This knowledge is
used in each piece of artwork created to carefully convey a
message, tell a story, or invoke a mood to the viewers. For
example:

• Reds tend to make you feel bold, passionate, bright.
  This warm color is usually associates with love, anger or
  courage.

- Orange is also a bright and warming color that is associated with youth and said to stimulate creativity and enthusiasm.

- Yellow is on the brightest side of the color spectrum and can give you a feeling of energy, joy, or hope.

- Green is entering the cooler side of the spectrum and is associated with nature, money, envy and health.

- Blue colors are the coolest side of the spectrum and can tend to give a feelings of confidence, trust, sadness, or calming.

- Purples are the transitioning color back into the warmer colors and can give a feeling of relaxation, sensitivity, power, or royalty.

- Blacks and whites are both neutral colors. This means they can take on any mood that yo assign to them If you think in terms of paint colors, when mixing a color with black it deepens and darkens the shade. When mixing a color with white, it lightens and brightens the shade.

When mixing three or more colors, you will either get a

shade of grey or brown depending on the exact mixture.

These are also neutral colors.

You also want to keep in mind the season your are

getting dressed in. The shade of a color really makes a

difference in mood and season. In the spring and summer,

light and bright colors are more prominent. On the other

hand, winter and fall colors are on the darker side. This can

very depending on where you live or if there is a holiday.

For example in the United States, Christmas is in the

winter time and the colors are traditionally a dark forest

green color paired with a bright bold red. Although these

colors are opposites, they pair well together and are

known to represent this particular season. Another

example is Easter. This holiday is in the spring and the

color scale associated with it are all light pastel colors and shades of white.These include light pinks, lavender, mint green, baby blue and soft yellows.

Textures in fabric operate in similar ways when it comes to seasons. The texture or feeling of a fabric is largely dependent on what the fabric is made of and the density of it. A staple all across the world and absolute timeless fabric is by far cotton. Cotton can vary in color, texture, and density. For example, the classic denim jeans are made of cotton and have a thick corse texture. Meanwhile, the classic t-shirt is also made of cotton but often has a light and smooth texture. Although the two are made with the same material, the different textures are used more commonly in different seasons. Full length jean pants may be too hot to wear in the middle of summer and are more common in the fall and winter, while a cotton t-

shirt may be too thin to wear alone in the middle of winter.
Its best that in warmer weather, you choose fabrics that is
lightweight, soft, and breathable such as light cotton, lace,
chiffon, mesh, linen, rayon, and polyester. Then in colder
weather, you choose fabrics that are heavyweight and
firmly woven together such as heavy cotton, wool, fleece,
cashmere, velvet, and leather

Fabric textures also carry moods with them. Fabrics
such as silk and lace are most commonly associated with
being sensual. This is why a lot of intimate wear and
pajamas are made from these fabrics. On the other hand, a
fabric like leather is looked at as being rugged or edgy.
This is why you see this fabric more often in jackets for the
fall and winter or associated with someone with an edgy
style.

This may sound a bit contradicting but because these tips on color, texture, and styles are just guidelines, any of these rules can be broken. Again, fashion is all about expression. That means there are technically no exact ways to dress. These are just the ideas that I find are the most commonly appreciated and loved by the majority. How you choose to break these guidelines is all a part of your personal style. Sometimes the goal is to stand out from the norm or get a memorable reaction out of your audience for entertainment. Think about how a typical clown at the circus is dressed. It breaks so many fashion rules! That's why it's not likely that anyone would wear that type of outfit in any other setting but to entertain.

This concept is also used for mascots, cartoon characters, and even anime. Well known characters such as *Goku* in *Dragonball* is known to have that signature orange jumpsuit that would probably look like an inmate outfit to someone who is unfamiliar. However, if you go to Comicon or a halloween party dressed as *Goku*, I'm sure many people with recognize the outfit when they see it. It was different from the norm, therefore it was memorable. This is why in some of the high-end fashion shows, there are pieces that to many people look completely ridiculous! This is still a part of fashion because not only did it get a reaction, but I'm willing to bet it was the most memorable of the show and drives more publicity. Publicity is great for business and sales. As far as the designer is concerned, mission accomplished!

Layaway and the Return Rack

Look at you! Popping with color, style on TEN and lifestyle is giving Luxury! Not to mention your confidence is at an all time high! You are successfully shaping your lifestyle and you are striving toward your own definition of success! This is definitely something to celebrate as I know it takes a certain level of boldness to step out into your own individuality. The work is not over just yet though. There is another part of this confidence building and lifestyle revamp that I don't think most people talk about. Internally you know you've changed for the better and worked really hard to get where you are, but there are some who may be confused at or indifferent towards this new you and new style. Once you've leveled up in life in any way, you're almost certain to experience moments that I like to call "layaway" or "return rack" moments. Let me explain.

Remember when I talked about the clothes I had as a kid in the beginning? Well, some of those clothes were purchased through layaway. The purpose of layaway back then was if you wanted to buy something, but didn't have the money to purchase it outright that same day. You would let the cashier at the store know you wanted to buy a particular item, and they would probably ask for you to pay a small portion of the total cost. Almost like a deposit or down payment. In doing so, the store would then set the item you wanted to buy aside and hold it for you until you were able to pay the cost in full. Afterwards when the full balance was paid, the store would then release the item to you for you to finally take home. I doubt too many stores do this anymore since today we have Buy Now, Pay Later options.

The point I'm making is, sometimes when you're going through life or presented with opportunities, people may put YOU on layaway. The people that didn't seem to be fully interested in you at first when you were still learning and growing, might start to reach out once you've started achieving more or leveling up your looks. You might see that random "Hey" text pop up after not hearing from someone in months. They might hit you with the "I see you're doing good! I'm so proud of you" once you've started seeing your success, but was never around when you were on the way up. And don't forget about the "I always knew you would do it" statement that comes from the very same people that may have tried to talk you out of or downplay your goals or ideas before. In the words of Mike Jones, "Back then they didn't want me, now I'm hot they all on me."

On an intimate level, this may look like the relationship you have with someone you like, but they've ghosted you up a couple of times or only reach out to you when they want something. They do just enough to keep you interested, but not enough to be consistent. As soon as you've changed up your style or maybe made changes to your body, here they come with all the love bombing. On the job, it may be you've spent years given it your all waiting for that raise or promotion, but the company keeps putting it off. As soon as you, start a second stream of income or start interviewing at different companies and no longer view this job as such a heavy priority anymore, here come all the talks of possible promotions or bonuses. This can even be that lifelong friendship you have where you are so familiar with each other and know intimate details about each other's lives. You can express all your anger and frustrations and they are with you all the way, but when it comes to your achievements, they are either nowhere to be found or it starts to feel like a competition. There could be little to no celebration for your achievements without a backhanded comment masked as a joke, or they start wanting to boast about all the achievements they've had instead.

These are all what I call Layaway moments. These people may have genuinely wanted to be around you in the beginning, but just didn't have what it takes to show you

your full worth or maybe just weren't all that interested in

you to be fully invested. As a result, you are put on hold.

It's just like an item being put on hold at the store. They

may come spend a little time with you here or

communicate with you there, but it seems very clear that

they don't take you seriously. You are not a priority to them

but they know if they come and make a small payment

with either time or conversation, you'll remain on hold.

Again, life is a journey, and we are human beings.

We make mistakes and don't always get it right the first

time. The idea is you want to allow space for others to be

on their individual journey, while being mindful not to be

taken advantage of. It's okay if other people are still getting

their lives together and make mistakes. What is not okay is

you just being dragged along as collateral damage. That is a sure way to destroy all the confidence and self esteem you've worked so hard to built up all this time. This happens all throughout life, but it might be more noticeable once you start leveling yourself up.

These type of situations can be tricky. On one hand, you might appreciate the fact that your hard work is visibly paying off and people are recognizing your value. On the other hand though, you may start to wonder why didn't they recognize your value to begin with? Well I would say that realistically, no one actually knows your full potential and capabilities except you. And even then, I'm sure that you too have surprised yourself a time or two when you did something you originally thought you couldn't. This should not be confused with clearly being treated poorly, but I do think that most times everyone underestimates

someone.

In this situation, I would reflect on how the

relationship with this person has effected me overall. You

can consider the pros and cons of having this person in

your life. As best you can, try to think of this logically

without letting your feelings cloud your judgment. For

example, say if you are in a relationship with someone and

they help out with providing for the household and maybe

the kids too, but they didn't seem to compliment you or

show appreciation for you often enough until you've had

your make over. I don't think this is an instance where you

were being taken advantage of. Sometimes a switch up in

your appearance is just what you need to keep your life fun

and energetic. On the contrary, if you used to be

completely ignored by someone you know but as soon as

you level up your money and get a new car so now

everyone wants to be your friend and ask for a ride every

other day, then you are probably just being taken

advantage of.

Ever so often, I believe it's beneficial to take a

mental survey of the people in your life. Consider if you

feel someone has put you on layaway and if it is a result of

getting caught in a routine that just might need to be

spiced up, or if you are actually being taken advantage of.

Maybe even you have put someone else in layaway. I'm

not saying you need to cut everyone off, but you may need

to review the relationship you have with this person. If you

realize that you have been getting constantly taken

advantage of, it might be a good idea to create some

space and distance yourself from this person for a while. If

a friendship, business partnership, or romantic relationship doesn't feel genuine and always costs you more than it gives to you, it might be a good idea to walk away. However, only you can decide that. This brings me to my "return rack" moments.

I think everyone has experienced at some point having to return something to the store after we bought it. As someone who has done this many times, I noticed it was sometimes hard for me to return certain items, even when I knew I didn't want it anymore. You spend so much time walking up and down an aisle or scrolling through Amazon to find something, just for you to finally get it and see that it wasn't what you thought it was. Similarly, parting ways with someone can be disappointing. You may have spent a lot of time and energy with this person so it makes it hard to leave. You would have to ask yourself if you would rather keep what you have knowing, it may not be the best option for you or release what does not serve you.

When you start behaving differently because you've changed your life for the better, old things won't fit anymore. The places you go to may not feel fulfilling, and conversations with the people used to hang around may start to feel draining. You may start to get called out for acting different, being accused of forgetting where you came from, or thinking you now know everything. This might even come from the people you dearly love. I know it's hard, but try not to get too discouraged. Everyone can't go where you were mean to go. This is your path in life and sometimes you have to be willing to start the path alone.

I've dealt with this myself where I had a close friend for almost 4 years. This person had seen me at my lowest times, and was present during some of my highest

moments. It wasn't until I started leveling up, doing

research, reading, and educating myself that this person

started to become what I felt was distant emotionally.

Anytime I would be excited to share something I learned,

my friend would reply with something like "Oh, I already

knew that." or "You're just now learning that?" Each time, I

would feel less and less excited to share the new

information that I learned with them. Then I started

noticing the side remarks and backhanded comments they

would make. After awhile, they would call me a smartass,

or say "You're just trying to be a goodie two shoes.." when

I went to volunteer in my community and even "I'm smarter

than you" when we would get into arguments. I didn't want

to accept it, but eventually I saw that my friend wasn't

exactly comfortable or aligned with this new path of self

growth that I had chosen for myself.

It was a difficult reality because this same person

had been there for me in my times of need. Even after

spending over four years around this person, I had to

decide to let them go. It was a painful decision but I knew

that because this person had a great deal of influence on

me, eventually their smart remarks and put downs would

lead me to either stop learning altogether or minimize

myself around them. I worked too hard to get to this point

let someone else on a different path deter what I feel so

passionate about. I also took a moment to observe this

person's own lifestyle, and noticed there were a lot of

things they did and were part of that I didn't agree with and

had caused me a lot of unnecessary problems and drama

in the past as a result. It reached a point where I felt there was more harm coming from the relationship than there

was help and it took a toll on my physical, emotional, and

mental health.

If you were waiting for a sign to let a person who

isn't aligned with you go, this is it. You've come too far and

worked too hard! Maybe later down the line you can circle

back and this person may be in a different space, but until

then its okay to stand on what you worked hard for. I've

also learned that once you start being willing to walk your

path, you meet new people on the journey that you can

walk alongside with. These are the people I met though my

fashion shows, at yoga, at dance class, when I took self

improvement classes and when I got out into my

community to volunteer. I know your tribe is out there too

and they will love the improved version of yourself because

they are most likely doing the same thing themselves.

Walk Your Runway

Although I love fashion and designing clothes, my mission and sole purpose for my brand is to build confidence. Take a moment to think about all things that lead you to where you are today. Think about all the ways you have grown and impacted the people around you. Earlier, I mentioned that I will go in-depth about the final stage of Maslow's Hierarchy of Needs since we've only discussed four out of the five stages. The final stage sitting at the very peak of the pyramid is Self Actualization. I saved this piece for last because if you take nothing else from this book, I hope you strive to achieve this stage in your own way, even if it has nothing to do with fashion. Self Actualization is your desire to become the best version of yourself that you can possibly be. This includes morality, spontaneity, acceptance, experience, purpose, and tapping into your inner potential. I believe this stage is the most powerful because this is the stage that has the most impact on those around you. This stage uses the other four in a way that gives back to their community and make it a better place. When others see you striving to reach your highest potential, it causes a movement within the community and can inspire the masses to do the same.

Operating in your highest level results in you helping others get their basic needs met with your abundance of food, shelter, clothing, etc. You can start businesses that will give security and employment to those needing income and safety. You can create communities of people who share the same values and will lift each other up that will create a sense of connection. You also have the power to awaken peoples creativity and and individuality. This is the level that all the great inspirational leaders and influencers of the world successfully operated in. This is the stage that creates change and progression across the globe within our human race. For me, this very book is my version of tapping into my final stage and my potential.

One of my favorite inspirational leaders and speakers is Jim Rohn. Mr. Rohn once said "Life is so risky, no one makes it out alive." This really stuck with me. It put things into perspective for me and made me realize that at some point, we all have an expiration date on this earth. The only thing that will be left is how you impacted the environment and the people around you. A teaching of Jim Rohn's discussed on how people operate and navigate through life within one of three categories. Dependent, Independent, and Interdependent.

The first is a childlike mentality where you are highly dependent on others. Think of when you're an infant or a young toddler who is dependent upon their parents for the physiological needs discussed in Maslow's pyramid. The child has no ability to think of how the parent is feeling what the parent needs or if they can fulfill their needs themselves. The child's needs getting met is completely dependent upon if anyone else around it decides to do so. Some adults still operate in this mindset. As an adult, this mindset can easily prevent you from ever getting your needs met, which will only result in you having a negative impact on those around you.

The second mentality is a person operating in independence. This means that a person is fully capable of relying on themselves to meet their own needs, as opposed to waiting for someone else to meet them for them. Think of a teenager who, as a child used to cry and beg for attention but now might seem to be annoyed or embarrassed by their parents involvement. They take great pride and being able to handle things themselves. This is a strong and healthy trait to have. However, this becomes an issue when this person begins to turn cold to others resulting in selfishness. This is where greed can grow and can also negatively impact those around you

Finally, the third mentality is interdependence. This trait is the telling factor of a true mature person. This mindset is a smooth transition from "I depend on you."

then "I depend on myself." then "You can depend on me."

This powerful statement means that you are not only

capable of relying on yourself to meet your own needs, but

you also take responsibility for others around you so that

they can depend on you. I believe this is the way of

reaching your highest potential of Self Actualization. I also

believe that this is how those who are wealthy and reached

a high level of success got to where they are.

These types of people are proactive and highly

effective in their lives. People like this don't wait for life to

happen to them, they go out and happen to life. A personal

goal for me is to strive everyday to become interdependent

while reaching the top of Maslow's pyramid. The vehicle

I've chosen to achieve this just happens to be through

fashion. I hope that within this book you feel my passion in

this and being of service. I also hope this book was helpful to you in some way. These are only some of the lessons

I've learned on my own personal journey as I look forward

to what else life has to offer me in the future. Even within

writing this book and revisiting some of my vulnerable

experiences, I find there is healing and sharing and in

community.

If you or someone you know, has ever struggled

with confidence I hope you now have some tools to use

and share to overcome little by little. I dedicate my fashion

brand to those who have ever felt less than or not

included. I want to thank both my parents Deena and Tim

for allowing me such creative freedom and trusting me to

carve out my own path. Thank you to my sister Morgan

who has always encouraged my creativity and desire for

entrepreneurship from the very beginning. I thank each and

every person that my journey has let me to cross paths

with, as each interaction has influenced who I've become today. If you ever need encouragement or just want to feel less alone, you can join my Sewciety on all my social media platforms.

Whether on Facebook, Instagram, YouTube, or TikTok, I strive to not only share fashion and sewing tips, but to track my ever evolving journey. If you have been inspired or encouraged in any way, I want to hear from you! I'm also curious to see all the creative styles and outfits that you come up with to enhance your own closet! You can find me on my website at www.aalichaw.com or you can tag me online at @aalichaw so I can share your experiences to encourage someone else too. Over time, I encourage you to revisit your inner fitting room as many times as you need to and reshape your style. When it comes to shaping both your lifestyle and your fashion style, you call all the shots. The world is your runway, so

walk your runway!